Exercise for Everyone

Sally Cowan

Contents

What Is Exercise?

Exercise is the movement of the muscles in the body in various ways. Exercise is good for everyone.

If we exercise often, our bodies become fit and strong. We will have plenty of energy to play sport and enjoy other activities. Exercise also helps us to think clearly, sleep well and even to make friends.

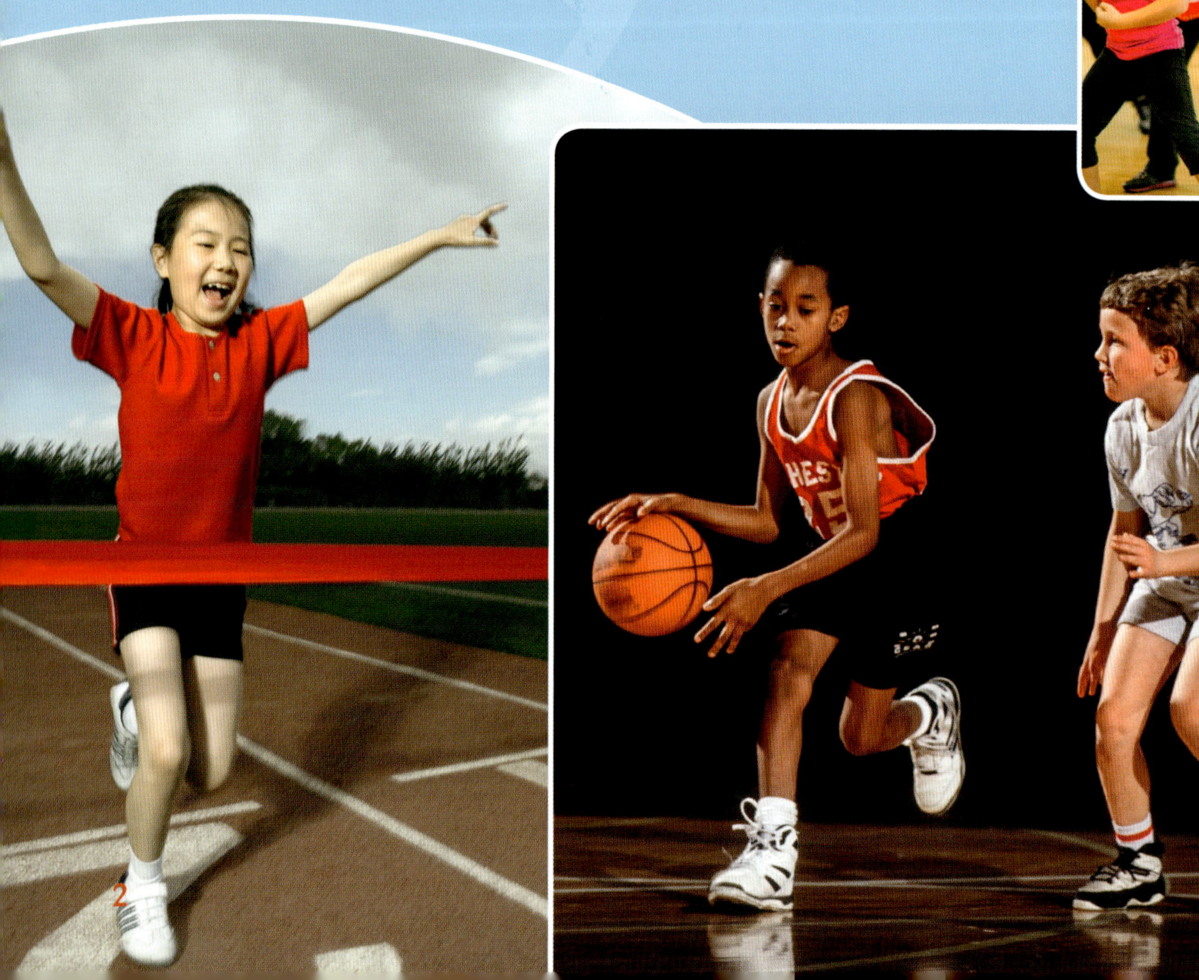

There are lots of different sports and activities that can **improve** our health and fitness.

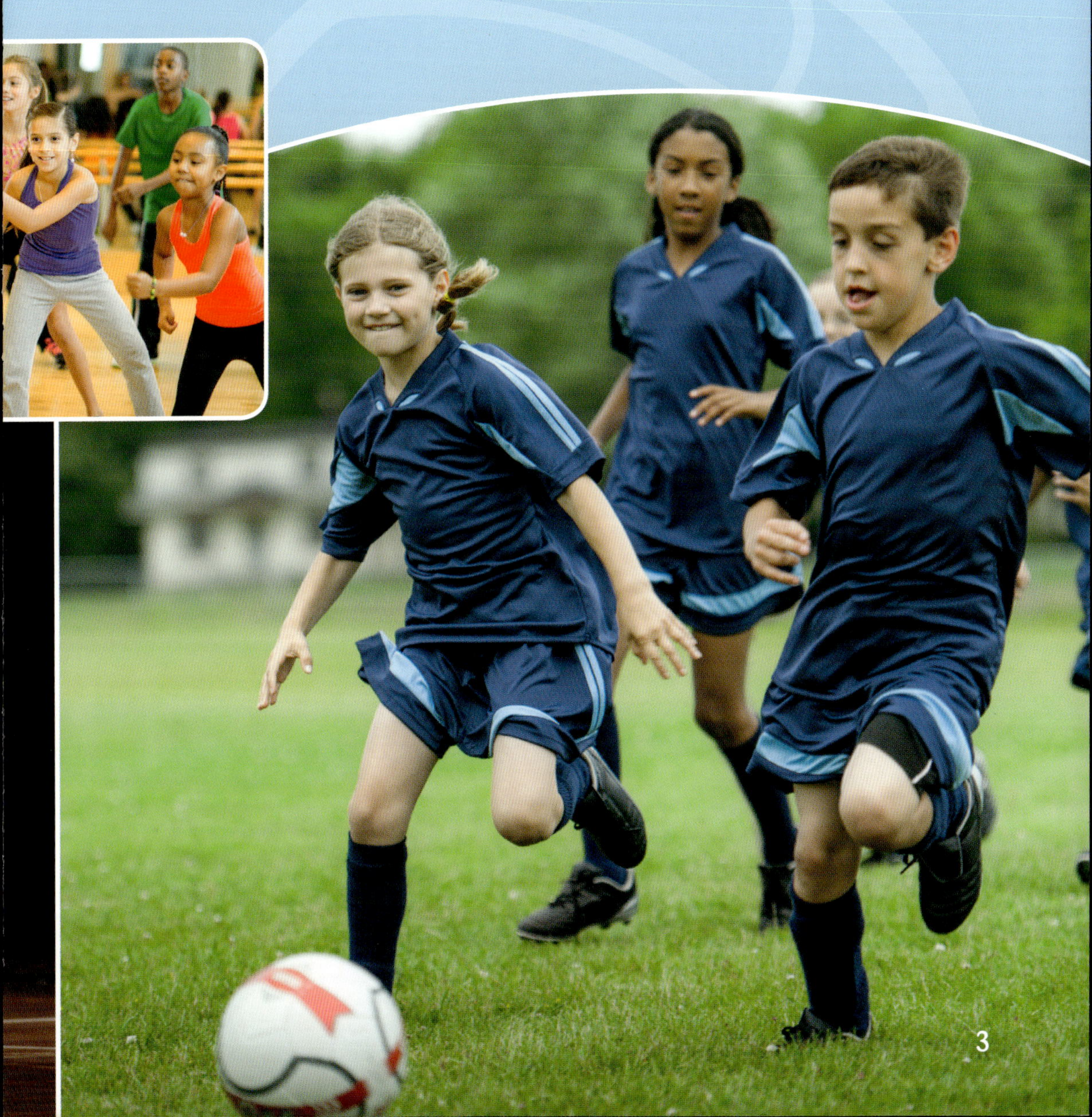

Exercise and the Body

Exercises with both fast and slow movements are good for different parts of the body.

When we run or move fast, we are doing **aerobic** exercise. This type of exercise makes our heart beat faster. Our lungs expand to take in more air, and our heart pumps blood quickly around our body. A strong heart and lungs are good for getting more energy.

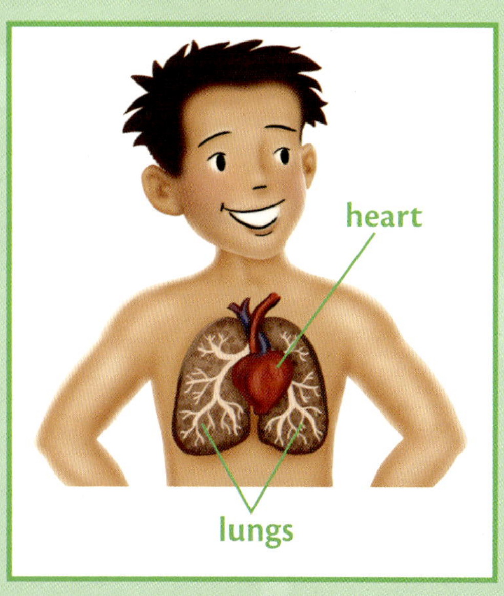

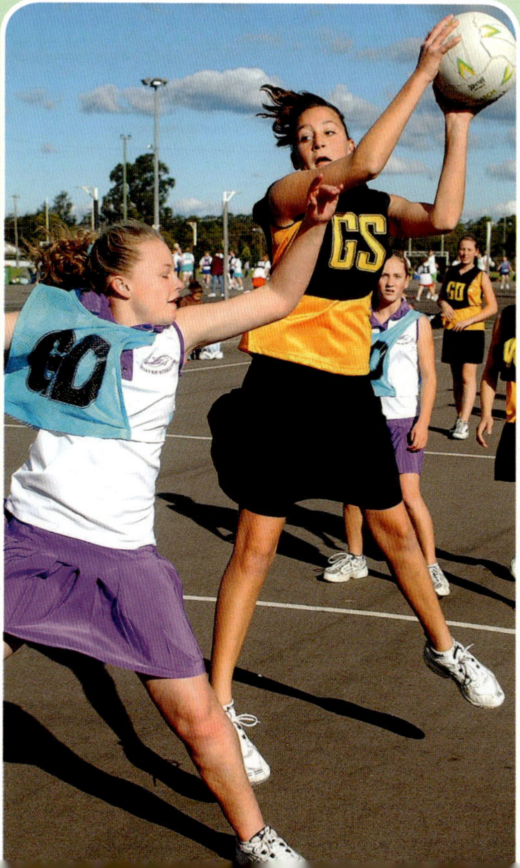

Many people enjoy taking part in aerobic sports and activities, such as football, netball and dancing. But any quick movements, even walking to school or playing with the dog, are suitable.

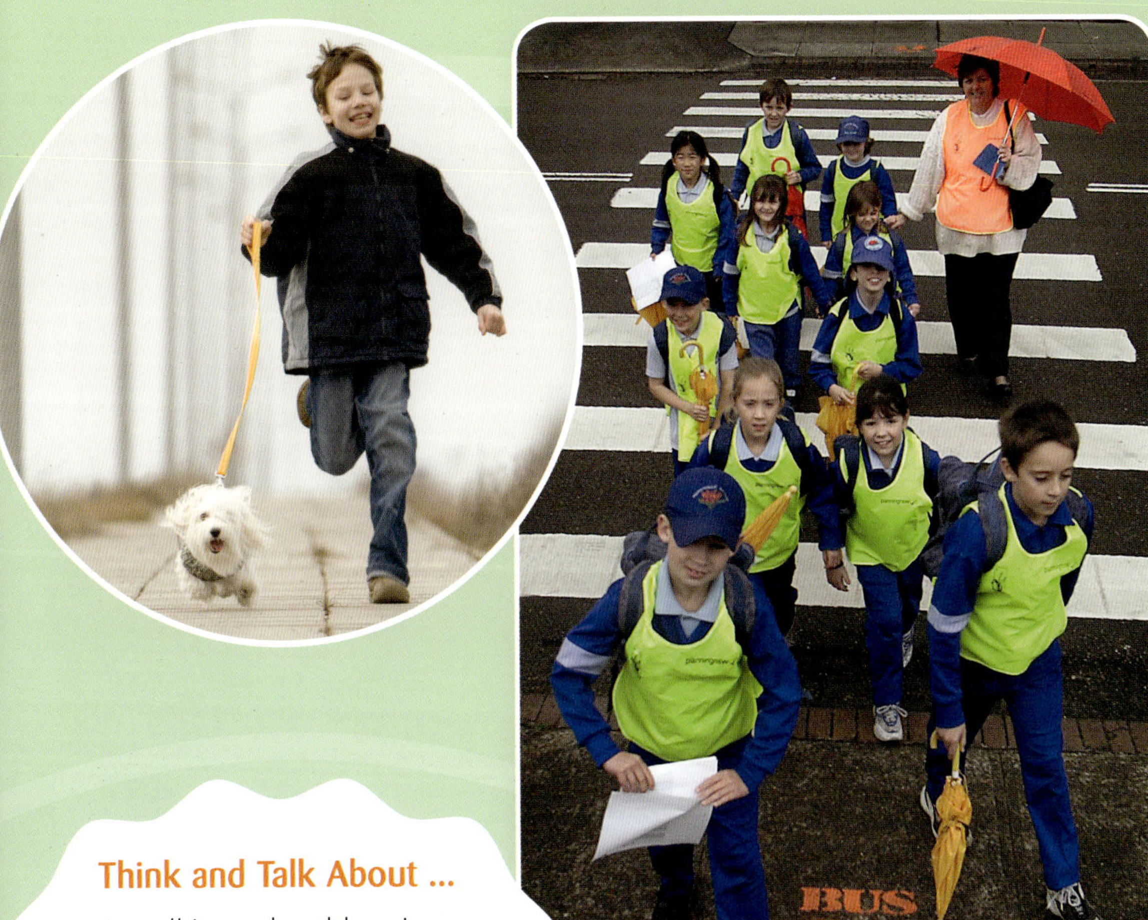

Think and Talk About ...

A walking school bus is a good way for young people to exercise every day.

Some exercises are good for making our muscles stronger.

Strong muscles allow us to control our movements well. In many ball games, the players must be able to catch or throw a ball. They also need to change direction quickly. The players can get better at their game by practising special **drills**.

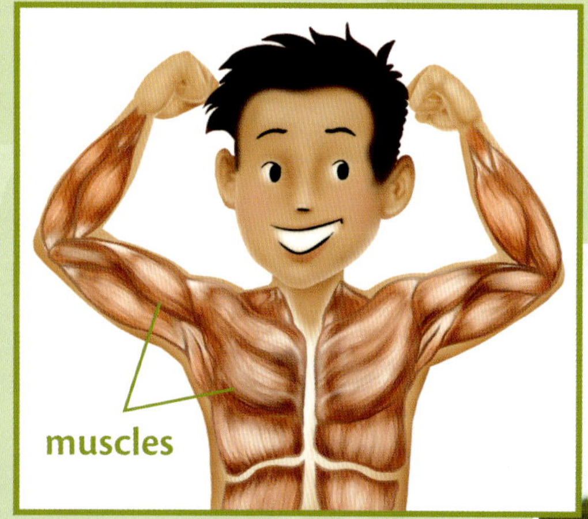

We should warm up our muscles **gradually** when we exercise. It is important to stretch them, too, or we might feel stiff and sore. Healthy, strong muscles also help us to stand up straight and keep our **balance**.

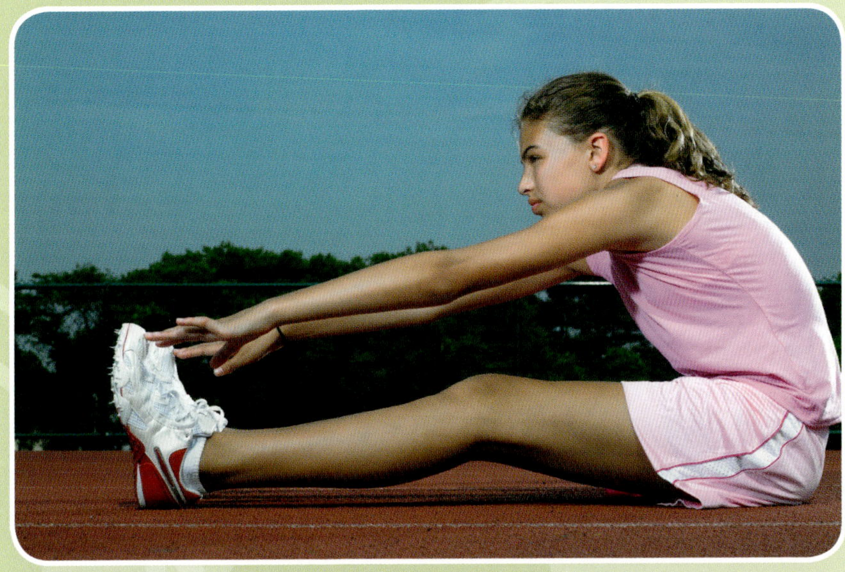

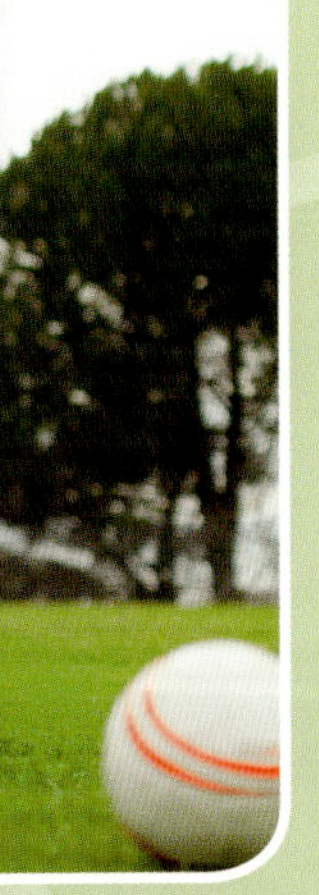

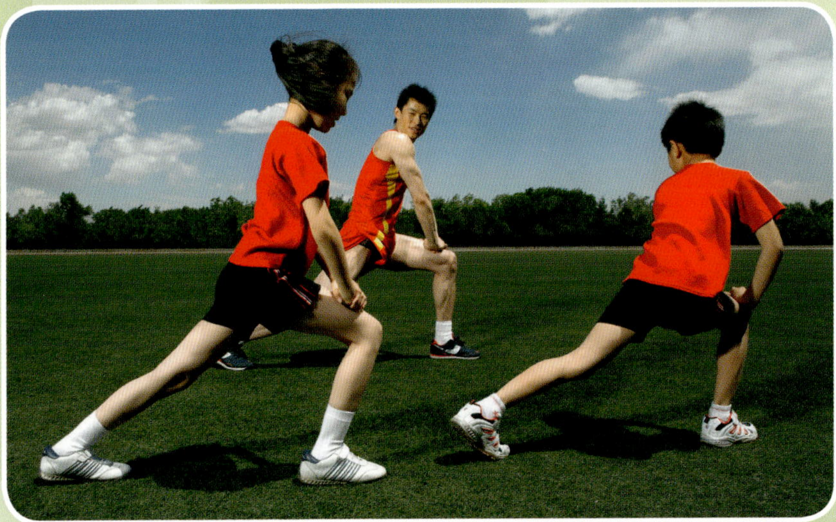

Thinking and Feeling

Exercise helps our brain stay healthy, too.
The brain is like a powerful computer that tells the body how to move, think and feel.

People who are fit and healthy can think more clearly than those who do not exercise. Having a healthy brain allows us to learn and understand things.

Healthy people often feel happy and full of energy.

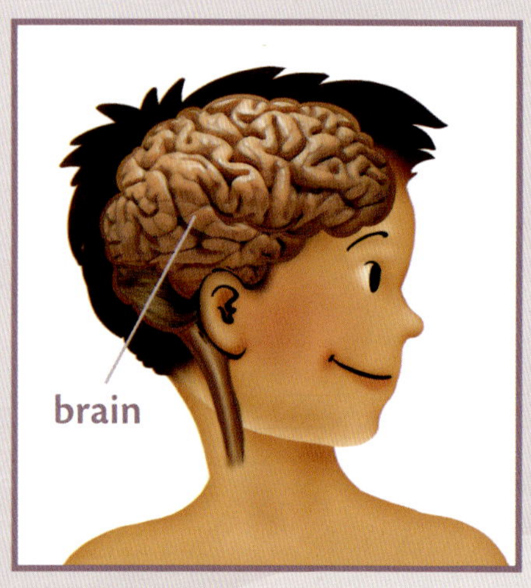

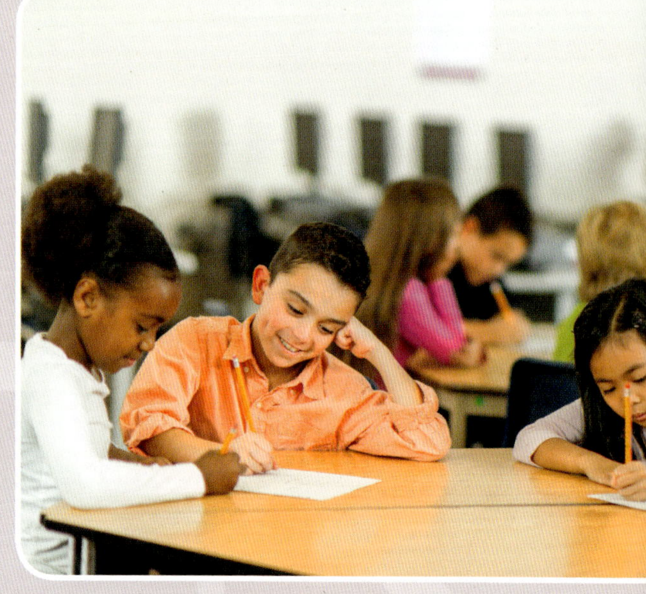

Sometimes, school students might have a difficult test or project to complete. Perhaps someone they know is sick. These kinds of problems can make them feel nervous or anxious.

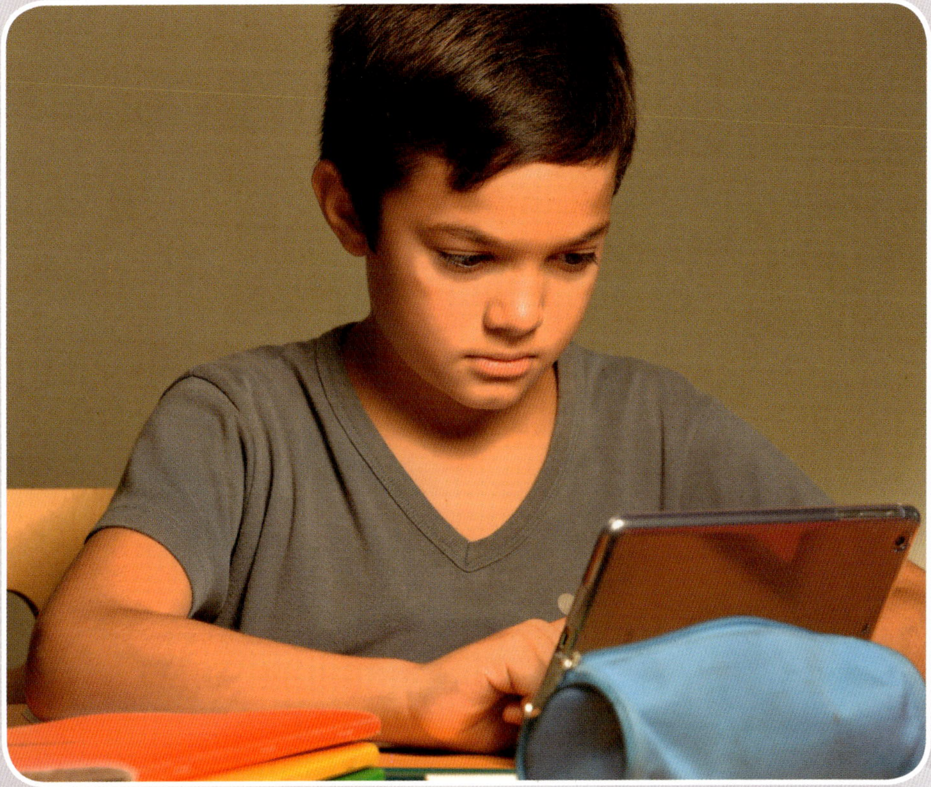

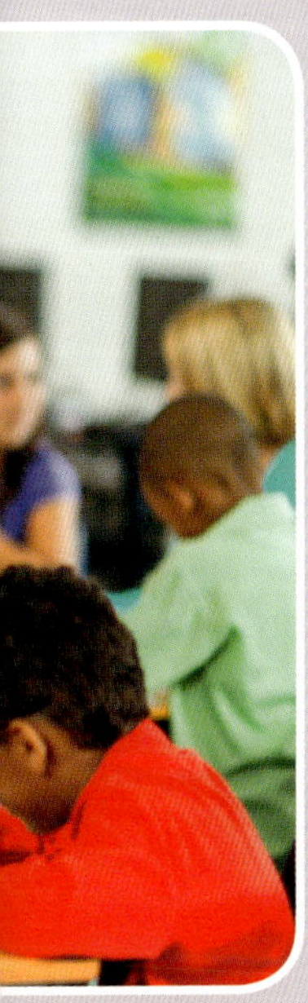

Regular exercise can help. Aerobic exercise makes us tired. Slow exercises, such as yoga, make us calm. When we are tired and calm, it is easier to sleep each night. Everyone needs a good night's sleep, so that they can be rested and ready for activities the next day.

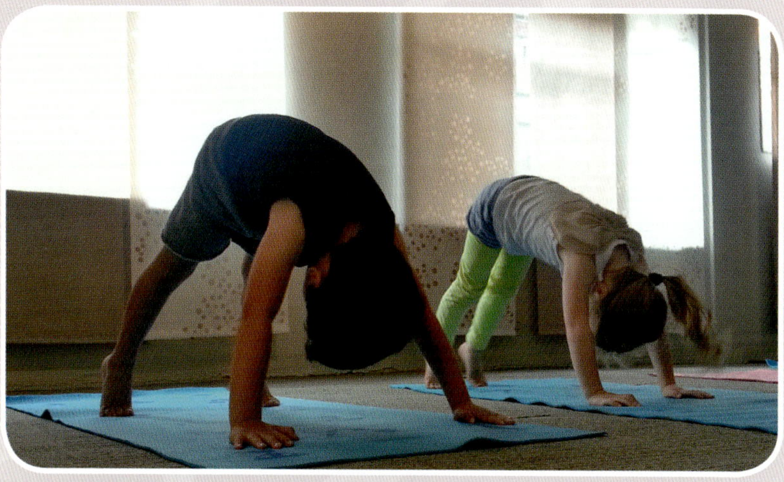

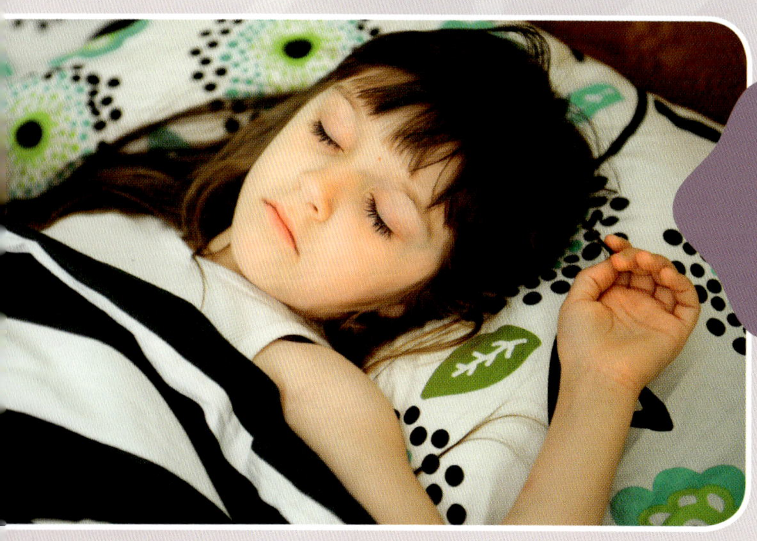

Think and Talk About ...

Students need between nine and eleven hours of sleep every night.

Teamwork and Friendship

Exercising helps people in other ways, too.

When we take part in sports or other activities, we can make new friends. In team sports, we learn to work together and think about others. Often, we have to follow rules, which teach us how to stay safe and be fair.

There are a lot of good reasons to exercise and stay fit.

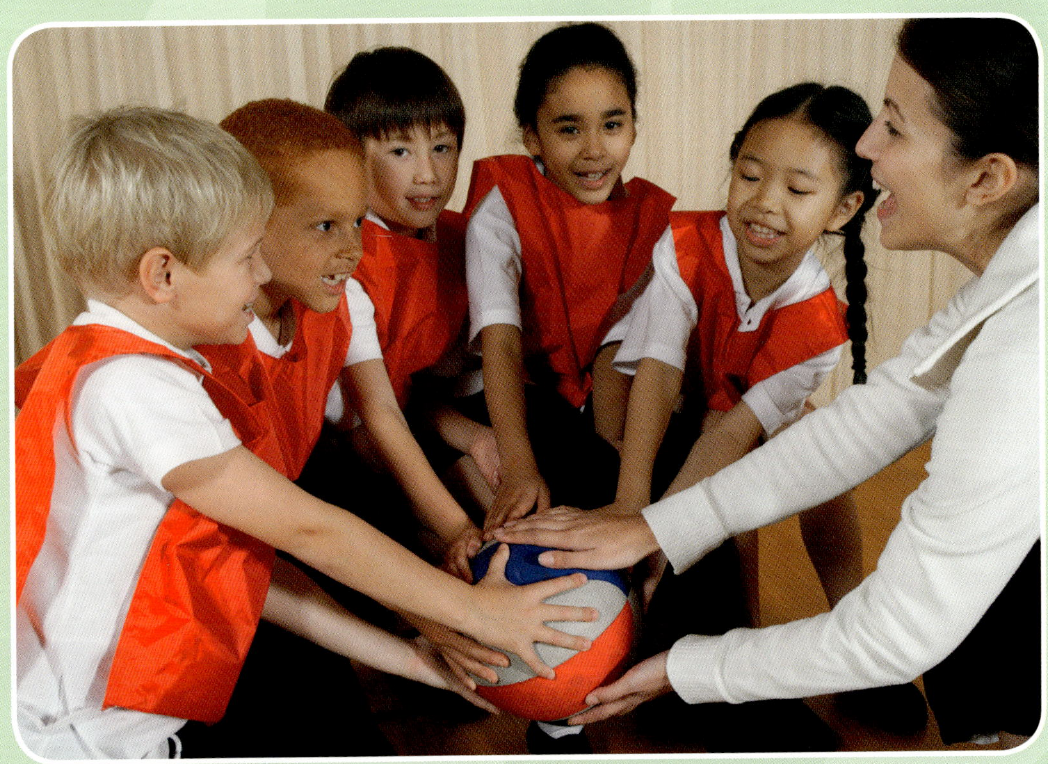

A Fitness Workout

Goal

To get fit by doing different exercises

Materials

You will need:

- comfortable clothing and sports shoes
- a clock or watch

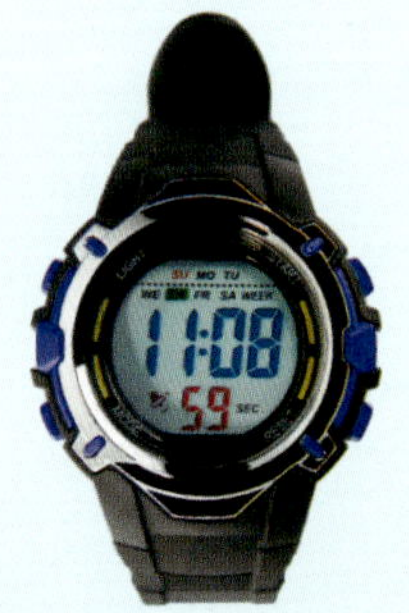

- a pen and some paper

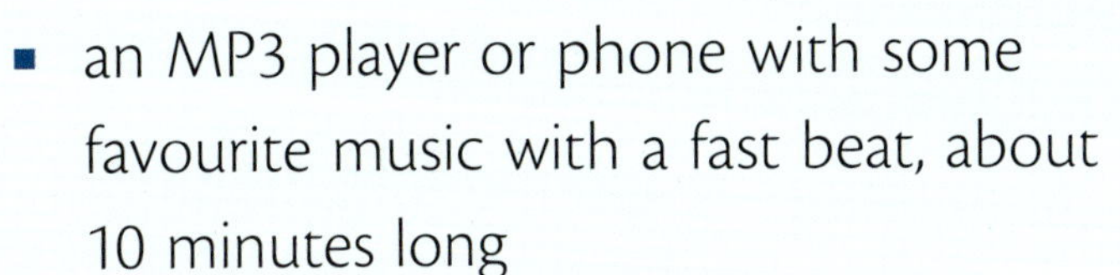

- an MP3 player or phone with some favourite music with a fast beat, about 10 minutes long

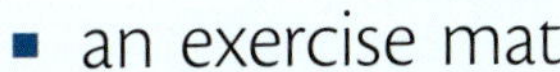

- an exercise mat

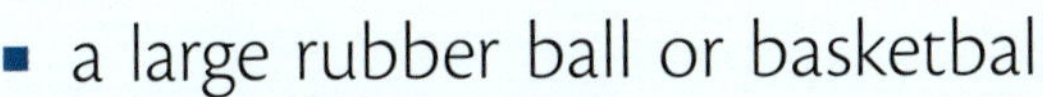

- a large rubber ball or basketball

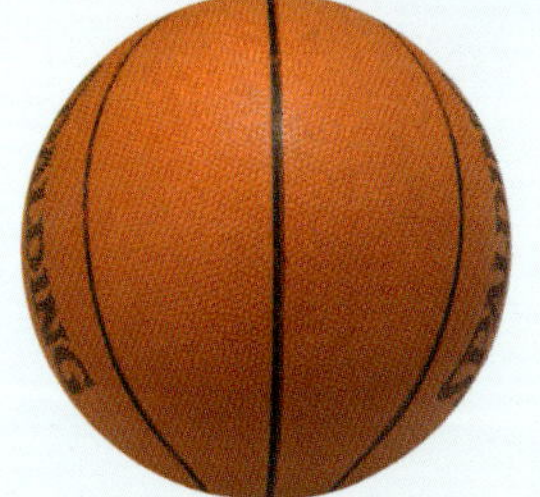

- a small beanbag.

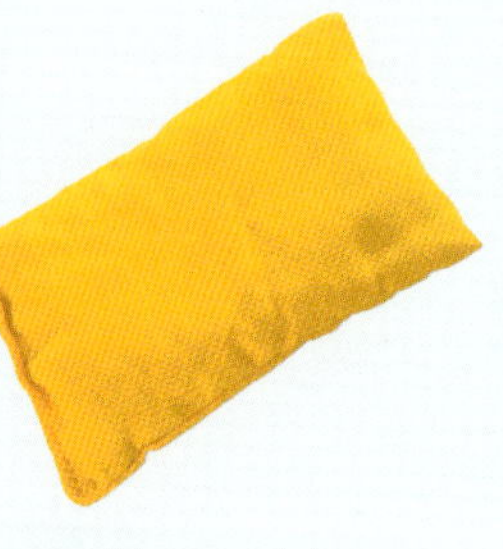

Think and Talk About ...

Young people need to exercise for at least one hour each day to stay fit and healthy.

Take Your Pulse and Warm Up

Steps

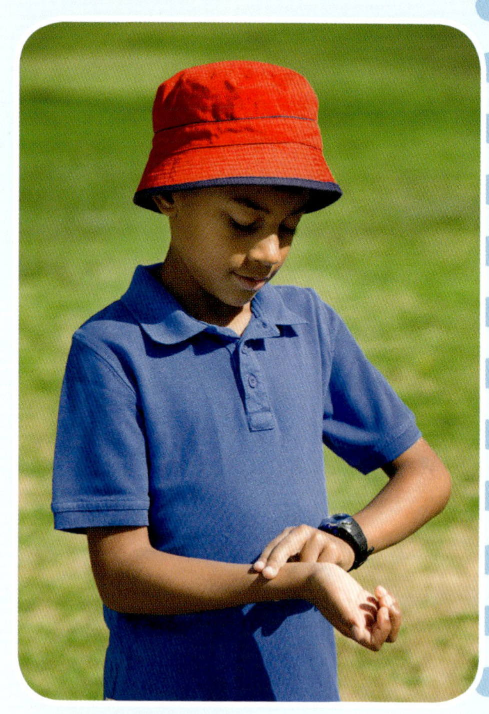

1. Use your index finger and middle finger to find your **pulse**. Place the tips of both fingers on the inside of your other wrist. Feel for the beat.

2. Look at the clock and count the number of beats for 60 seconds. This is your pulse rate.

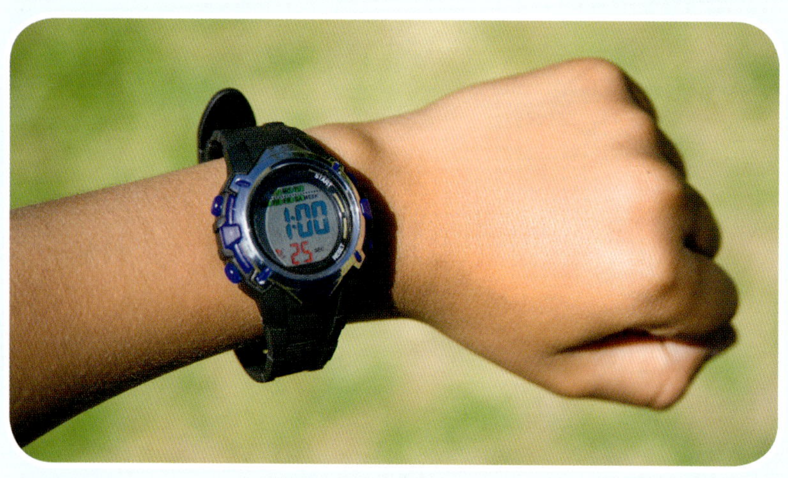

3. Write your pulse rate on the paper.
4. Start your warm-up by marching on the spot, then jogging, for 90 seconds.
5. Take your pulse again for 60 seconds and record the number of beats. Your heart will now be beating a bit faster.

Pulse rate
before exercise: 90 beats/minute
after exercise: 130 beats/minute

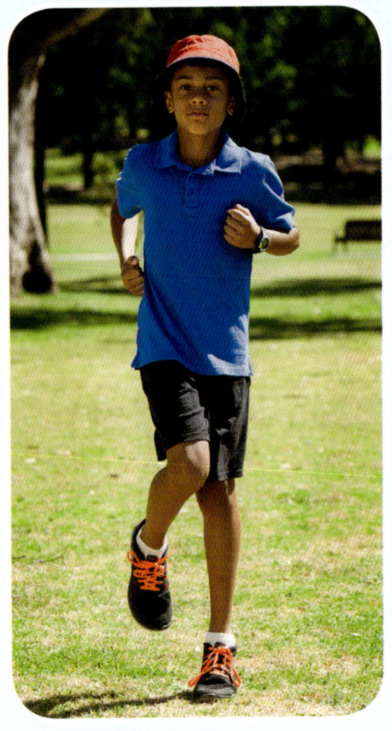

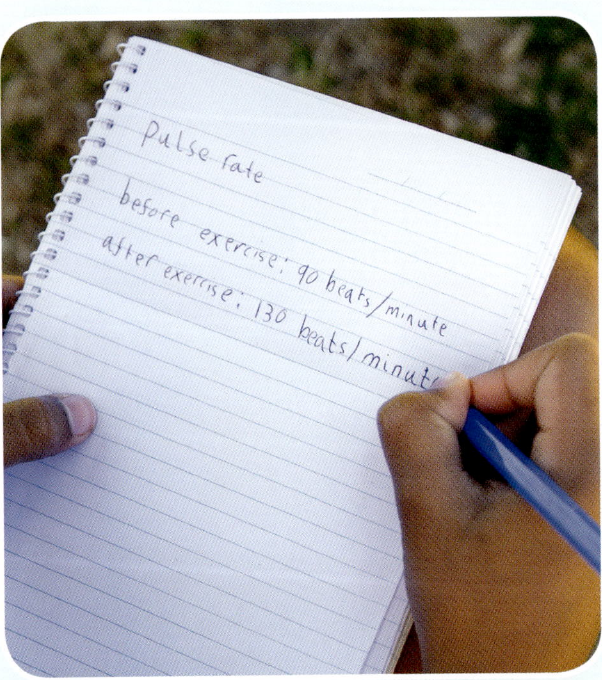

Think and Talk About ...

Take your pulse during a vigorous workout, to see the difference in your heart rate.

Aerobic Exercise

Steps

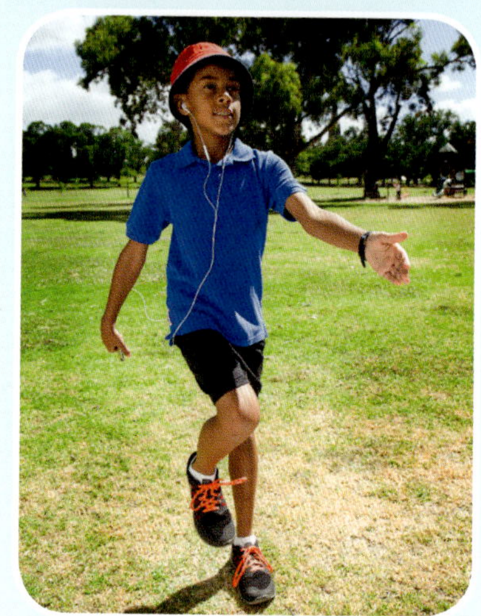

1. Turn on the music and march on the spot for about one minute.

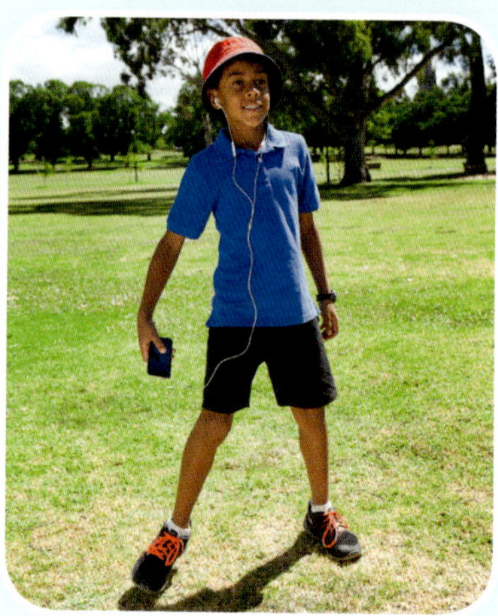

2. Stand up straight, with your knees **slightly** bent. Step one foot to the side and tap the other foot next to it. Repeat from side to side, 20 times.

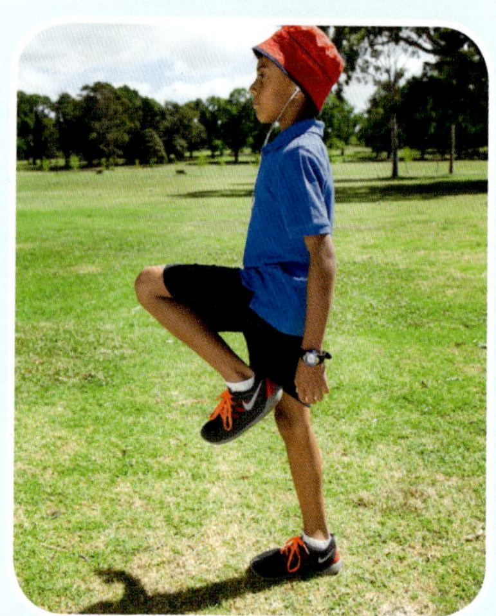

3. Do 20 knee lifts for each leg, raising one knee at a time. Let your arms drop down when you raise a knee, and lift them up when you put your foot down.

4. Do 10 star jumps.

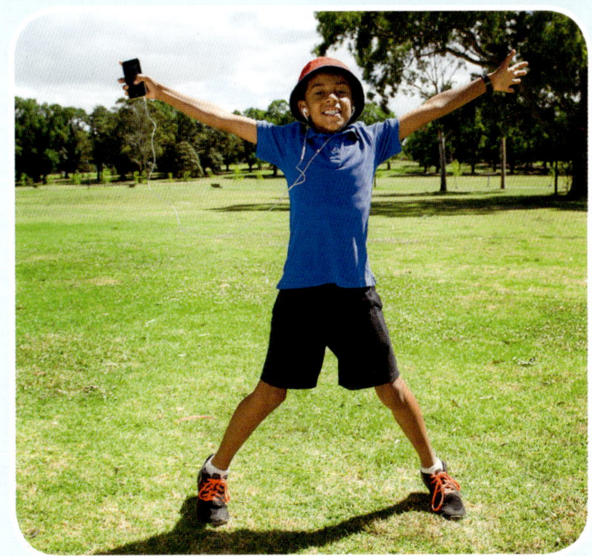

5. Make up some of your own dance moves for two minutes.

6. Repeat Steps 2 to 5 until the music has finished playing.

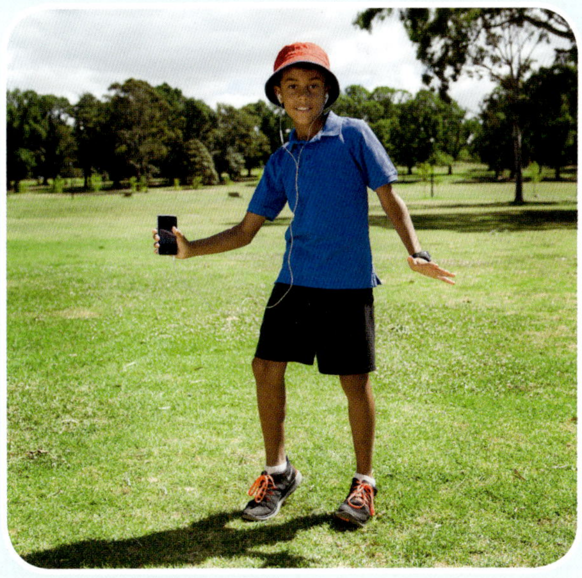

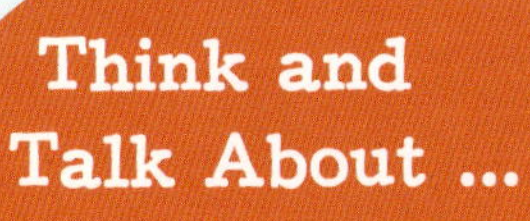

Aerobic exercise will make your heart beat much faster.

Muscles: The Perfect Push-Up

Steps

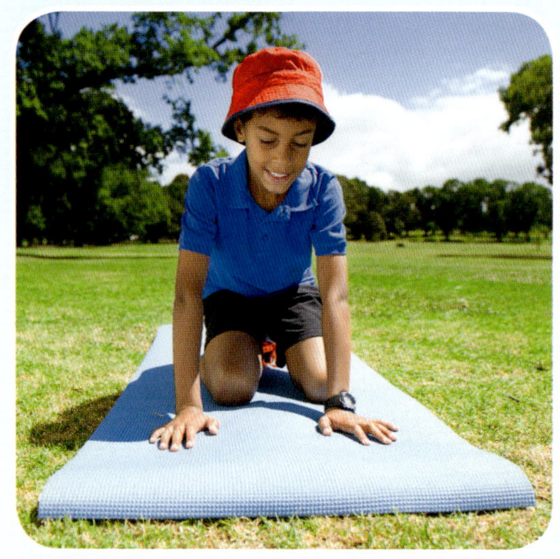

1. Kneel on an exercise mat. Bend over and place your hands on the mat.

2. Make sure your hands are below your shoulders. Have your fingers facing forwards. Your knees should be on the ground below your hips. Look down at the mat.

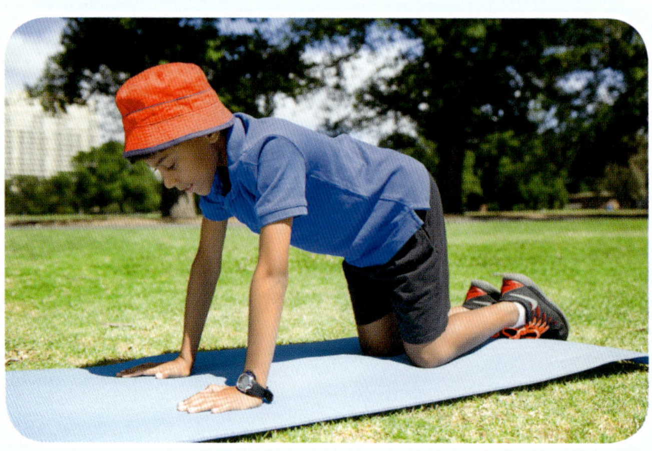

3. Keep your neck and back straight. Slowly bend your elbows and lower your chest towards the ground. Don't touch the ground.

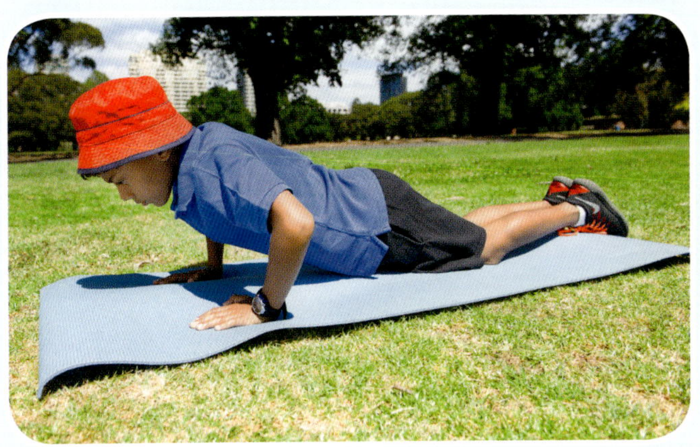

4. Straighten your arms again and push your body up.
5. Repeat the push-up four more times.

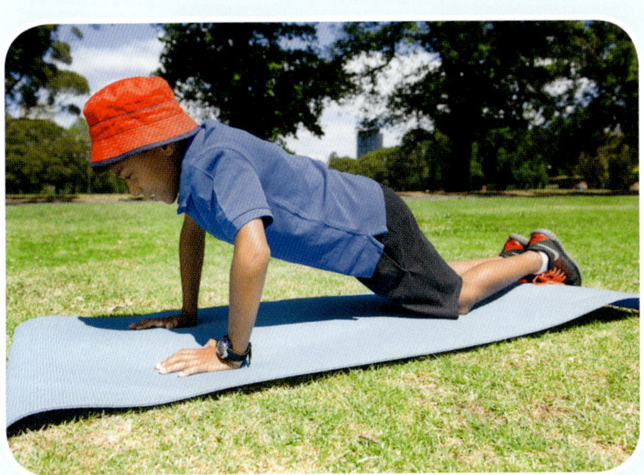

Think and Talk About ...

People must be careful not to lift weights that are too heavy for them, or they might hurt their muscles.

Control: Ball and Beanbag

Steps

1. Take the ball and bounce it several times on the ground. Bounce it with one hand and then with the other.

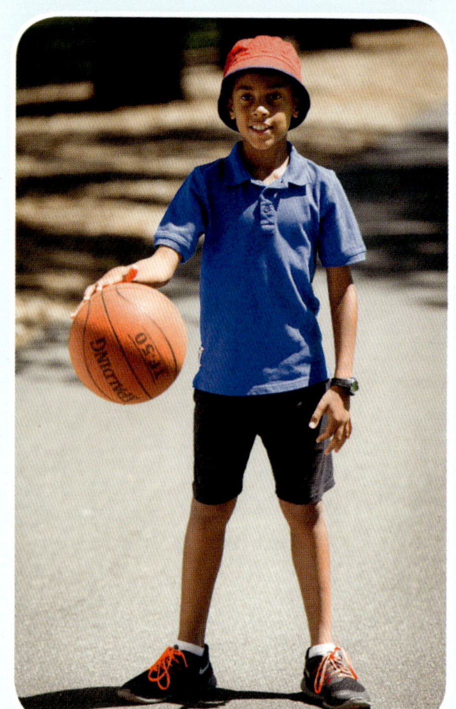

2. Begin to walk or jog in a straight line, while bouncing the ball with one hand.

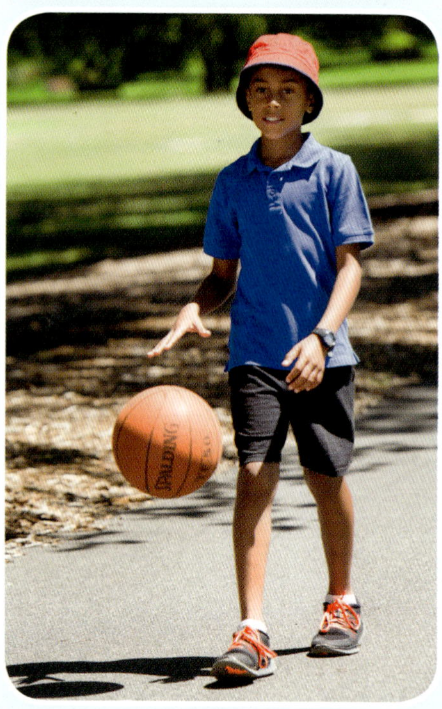

3. When you have moved forward about 10 metres, turn around and come back again.
4. Repeat this exercise using the other hand.

Think and Talk About ...

Ball games are easier to play when using both hands.

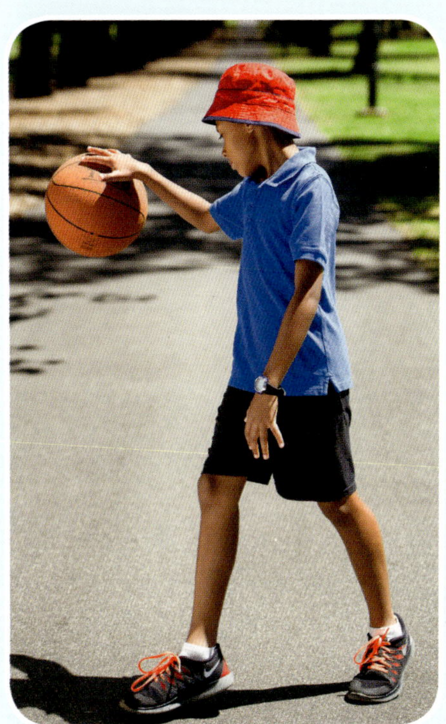

5. Place the beanbag on your head. Stand up straight and tall.
6. Walk carefully, keeping the beanbag on your head.
7. Move forward about 10 metres, then turn around and walk back again.

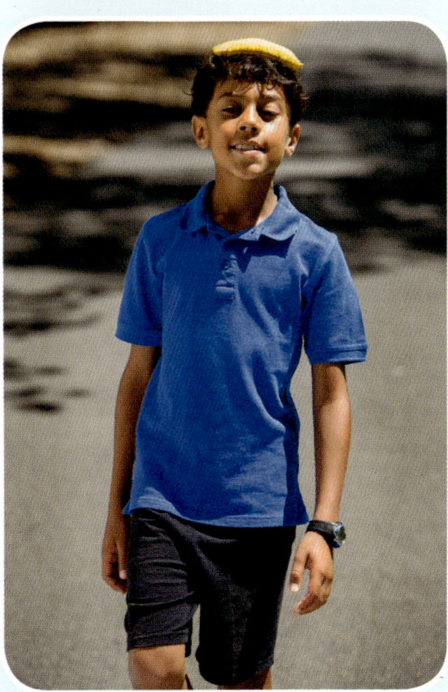

Yoga: Plane Pose and Cat Stretch

Steps

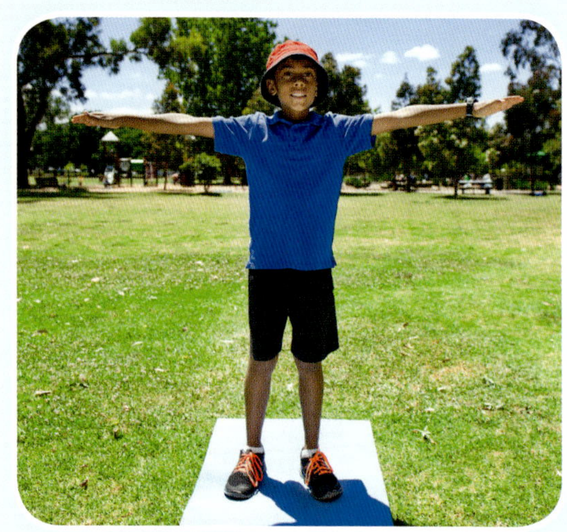

1. On the exercise mat, stand up straight and stretch your arms out to your sides, like the wings of a plane.

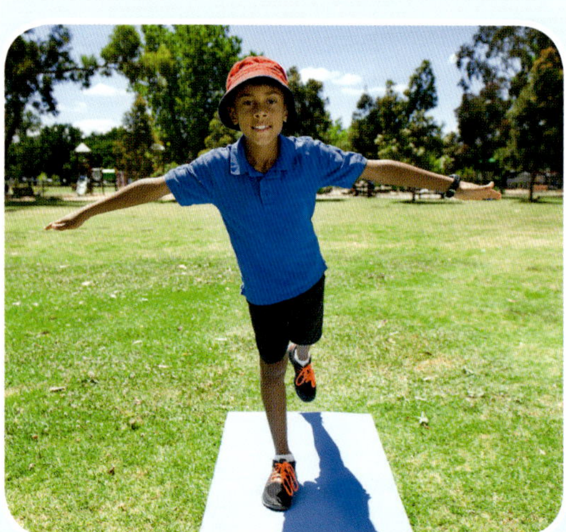

2. Lift your left leg up behind you. Balance on your right leg and lean your body forward. Stay still for as long as you can.

3. Repeat with the other leg.

4. Finish with a cat stretch. Get down on your hands and knees.

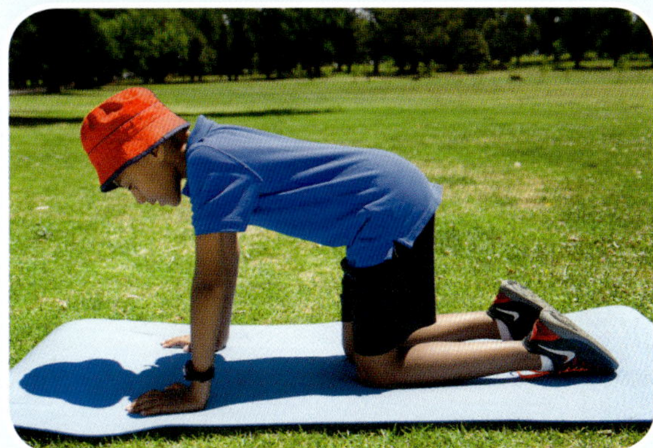

5. Take a deep breath in. Then, breathe out as you stretch and round your back up high. Meow like a cat as you breathe out!

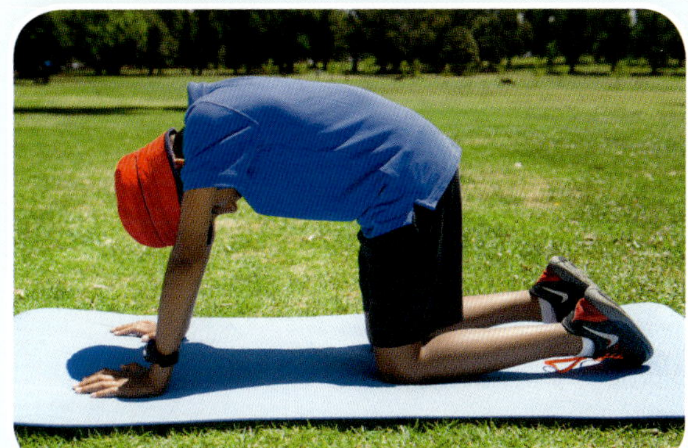

6. Now, breathe in as you look up and lower your stomach towards the floor.

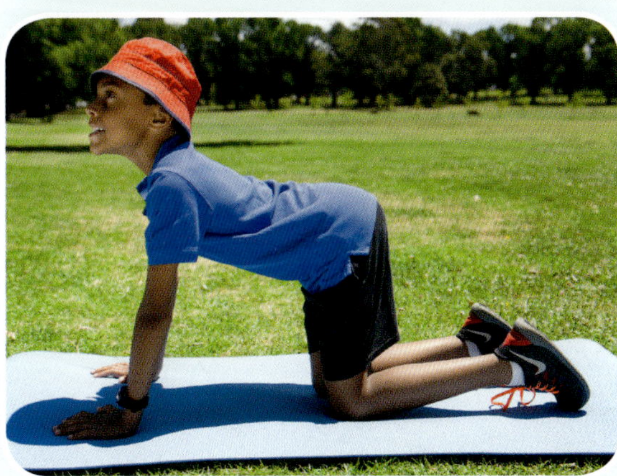

Think and Talk About ...

Some yoga exercises have the names of animals.

Glossary

aerobic *(adjective)* taking a lot of air into your heart and lungs

balance *(noun)* steadiness

drills *(noun)* activities that are repeated many times

gradually *(adverb)* beginning slowly, then getting faster; not quickly

improve *(verb)* to get better at something

pulse *(noun)* the heartbeat felt through the skin

slightly *(adverb)* just a little

Index